MARK SOBEY

Christmas At Dad's

A guide for single and divorced dads

This book was professionally typeset on Reedsy.
Find out more at reedsy.com

Contents

Introduction

Introduction:

I'm writing this as a helpful guide for single or divorced dads to navigate raising their children successfully.

The title "Christmas at Dad's" is a statement of what I think about when I think of my children. This was and is always a cherished memory for me on a yearly basis.

A brief background about myself. I am a divorced dad with three wonderful children; two daughters and a son. I've been divorced for around twenty-three years now and all my kids have grown up and have lives of their own.

What we will be discussing in this book is how they got to where they are today. The journey that they and I took to get here to this point in our lives. There are a lot of negatives and positives when you are a single dad raising three children, but for the purpose of this book, we are going to concentrate on the positives. Number one rule: be optimistic.

1

Chapter 1: In the beginning

The number of single father households has grown from 1.5 million in 1980 to 3.5 million. This is one of the fastest growing populations in America. There is a need to help single fathers as much as single mothers. But what is most important is the well being of the children. There are over 23 million children living in single-parent households in the US. That's an astounding number.

Your children can go through a range of emotions during and after the divorce. Most of the normal emotions are anger, loss, sadness, anxiety, and confusion. Children may feel angry that their parents are divorcing. Loss because they don't have both of their parents together anymore. Sadness that this is happening to them and this could lead to some depression symptoms you need to look out for. Anxiety about the major changes in their everyday life. Finally, confusion; how did this happen? Is it my fault?

For the most part, these emotions are short-term. I have three children who were approximately eleven, ten, and five years of age when my divorce happened. They experienced different emotions because of their age differences, which means sometimes you're dealing with more

2

than one issue at a time. This can be overwhelming at times. Again, number one rule, stay optimistic.

Some of the things you can do to help your children get through this process are communicate with and listen to them. Hear them out on their feelings about the situation and discuss it in a positive manner, like the bright spots of the situation. At this time early in the process, don't burden them with the emotions you are going through. Look for outside support for that, like your family, friends, or a professional. Try to explain how things are going to change and what things are going to remain the same. Spend as much time as you can with them doing activities and show them plenty of love and warmth. Give them hugs and kisses!

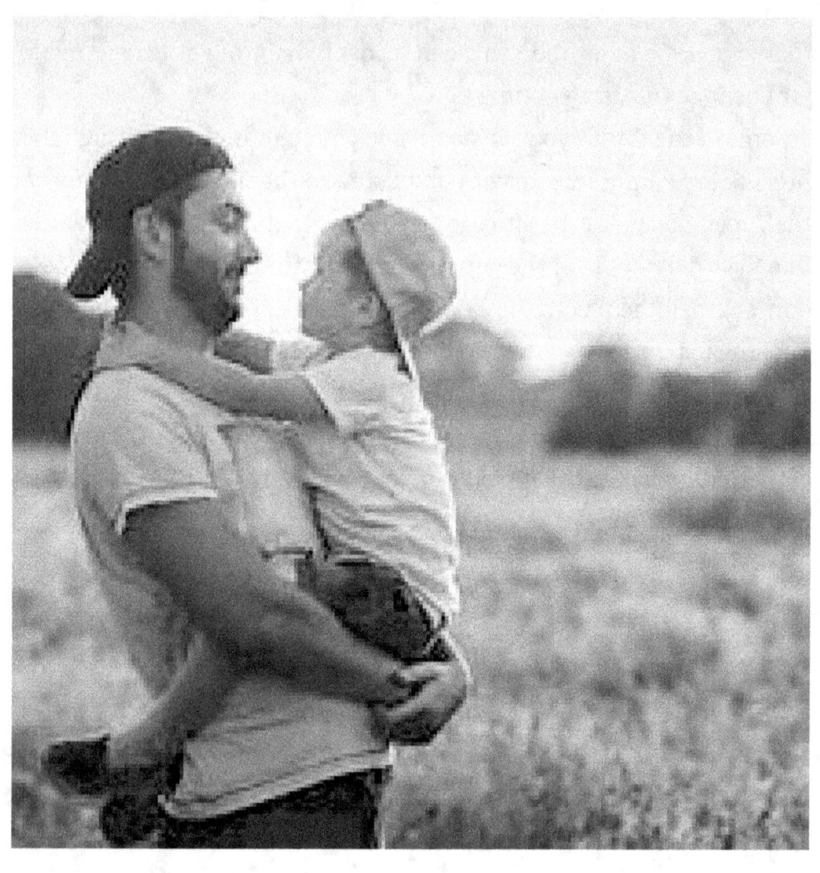

2

Chapter 2: Co-parenting

If you are getting a divorce, you need to learn how to co-parent with your ex-wife. This is how my experience began. When my wife served me papers, we were living apart and both spending time with our children. My children were in the car when I found the divorce papers in my sun visor. My ex had left them there when she transferred the kids to me. So I opened this envelope in the car in front of my children because I didn't know what it was. Everything became very real for the kids and me at that moment. What really made me want to be a major part of my children's life is the fact that all of them looked at me sincerely and said they wanted to live with me. I decided to fight for custody, only 50/50, so I could be in their lives as they grow up. Thank God I received 50/50 joint custody. It was a changing point in my life.

Parenting can be nurturing if both the mom and dad work together. Luckily we were able to do that and put the kids first. You must communicate with each other in a pleasant way, particularly in front of the children. Both parents set mutual boundaries for the kids and bring enjoyment and happiness into their lives. If possible, still do some activities with mom, dad, and children. That's not always going to work for some, but it does show the kids unity and support. You must learn how to not resent your ex. Put on an act if needed for the children's sake.

Some things to avoid to create a more positive situation. Don't use your children as go-between and don't criticize their mother in their presence, no matter how you feel about her. Remember, this is for the children. Make sure you leave an open line of communication with your ex so the kids are not trying to get away with shenanigans. They will sometimes try using the trick of saying, "Well, Mom lets me," or vice versa. Also, don't let your ex-wife use you for material things, emotional things, or monetary things by using any residual feelings you may still have for her. If you both work together in a positive way, this can go a long way to help your children through this process and the rest of their lives.

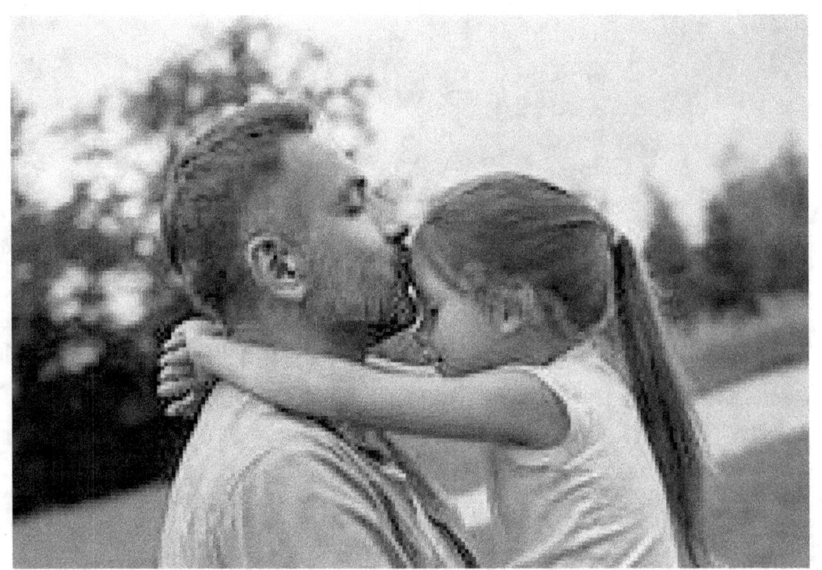

3

Chapter 3: Bonding

Besides the turmoil in a single father's life, there are way more memorial times now and ahead. It's important to try and bond with your children on a personal level. Show your love often and tell them you love them. It's important for their emotional development to ensure that they are loved unconditionally. A child does need structure in their life though. It's important they know the rules and consequences of breaking those rules. It's also important that you and your ex are on the same page if you're divorced.

It's also important for you to connect with them by listening to their thoughts and feelings. Always let them know you are there for them and assure them you will always be. Make sure you set time aside for your children. Trust me, I know it's difficult when you are working a full-time job and more hours than most. There are always things you can make time for. Have family dinners together, cook together. We even washed clothes together. We also played together though, and that is also important to their development. It could be as simple as playing basketball in the driveway with your son and maybe his friend in the evening. Maybe singing karaoke with your daughters in the living room.

All my children enjoyed playing video games and I loved that part of being with them. I've always played video games since I was a child, all the way to Pong by Atari.

If you have more than one child, spend individual time with each and do what they like to do. Let each of them know they are special. You can read to them or with them, color with them, do school projects with them. We watched a ton of Disney movies together and I think I loved them as much as the kids did. I may have slipped in some movies that maybe we shouldn't have been watching, like "Die Hard" and "Deep Blue Sea."

Help them with their homework. It may make you a little smarter too. Don't make the mistake I did though. Instead of learning how to take advantage of new tech every year, I shamefully would just hand the phone, computer, or gadget to one of my children to fix or make work.

You want to be there for your children and you want them to have fond memories of you and their time with you. Have fun together, play board games, play dolls, have a tea party. Just spend time with them doing whatever they want, and make sure you and your kids are smiling or laughing during your time together. Remember, positive attitude; it will grow on them.

There is no way to guarantee your children will remember everything, but the more good things that happen, the more they will remember and the better they will turn out as human beings. Many things that they really remember are spontaneous things. I bought my children and I a family pass to Six Flags and sometimes I would just pick them up from school and go ride roller coasters during the week.

Make sure you go to as many of their activities that you can attend. Baseball games, basketball, football games, all my son. I attended high school games that my son didn't play in just to watch my daughters in marching band for half-time shows. I made a point to make sure my kids participated in some type of school activities or team-building experiences. I can remember so many concerts, dance recitals, school musicals or plays, debates, little girl cheerleading, and tennis matches. I was always there to encourage my children and I enjoyed it. Those are particularly bonding moments when they see you there. Try and be a huge part of their lives so they remember that part of their lives. Just be there for them!

4

Chapter 4: Creating memories

I believe firmly in doing activities together that they will have fond memories of the rest of their lives. Family activities are important and necessary for many reasons. Family activities strengthen emotional bonding between family members. Why is this important? It helps the family members feel valued and supported, including yourself. It builds a strong foundation for emotional wellness. Spending time together as a family can help your children's overall mental well-being and provide emotional health. Family time can also reinforce your family's self-concept, their family history, cultural history, values, and beliefs. Doing activities together can give your children a sense of stability and security. When family members spend time together through activities, you're sharing experiences that will bond you and create memories they may remember the rest of their lives

There are countless activities you can do as a family. Many are budget-friendly as well. You can go on hikes together, have picnics together, partake in game nights and movie nights. There are so many, it's impossible to name them all. So I'm just going to go through what my children and I did to spend time together. My family likes to travel, so we did a lot of trips, usually during the summer. I think this goes back to my childhood and our family trips. Anyways, some of the activities were just taking my children to the public pool. As I mentioned earlier, we loved Six Flags and water parks. First trip I remember we took together was a week at Disney World. We didn't have much money at that time, so the four of us bunked together in the same small hotel room at, I believe it was called, the Rock and Roll Hotel. They had different themed hotels at that time. I purchased a family park pass, which got us into four enchanting theme parks and two water parks. We had so much fun trying to do everything in a week. Unfortunately, we missed out on dinner with the princesses. You have to book that far in advance. Instead, we had dinner with Winnie the Pooh and Tigger too, the whole gang. This was mainly for my youngest daughter who was probably around six or seven at the time. Amazingly, we all enjoyed it thoroughly. These are all the great memories that I have. I hope my kids do as well.

As the kids grew older, we did different things. We went to concerts together. Once we drove down to South Padre Island off the coast of Texas. They have beautiful white sand there. We brought my sister's son with us, who was the same age as my son. My children spent a lot of time with their cousins from Houston. They were in the same age group. Anyway, the activity I remember the most was taking surfing lessons at a place called "The Jettes." Probably the only place you can kind of surf in Texas. We were actually surfing together. Well, some surfing, mostly falling. Great memory!

We have done so many other things together. The reason I'm telling you about our adventures is so you can have some alternatives to the same old activities they talk about in other books. My youngest daughter and I took a trip together to New Braunfels for river tubing with one of her friends. We also traveled to Riviera Maya, Mexico together. My son, youngest daughter, and I spent time at South Beach, Miami as well. We've actually been twice, once for a wedding and once for vacation. My oldest daughter and I went to Jamaica together. These were all trips and things we did as they were growing up.

The trips didn't stop there, though. I still to this day try to plan family trips together. Our latest adventures include, in order, traveling to Colorado and renting a condo. We hiked, played golf, and white water rafted down the Royal Gorge. That was about four years ago. Two or three years ago, we went to Spain. This time with my youngest daughter and her husband and my son and his wife. The latest memory was spending 12 days in Italy. We went to my sister's daughter's wedding and stayed longer to see the rest of the country. Vienna was awesome!

There are so many other trips we took, like golf trips with my son and weekend trips with everyone. I know some of the things can be expensive, but you can start off small with day activities or weekend trips camping. As you grow with your children, you can really experience some great times together and build better memories. Oh yeah, we all four went to Hawaii together. Can't forget that one.

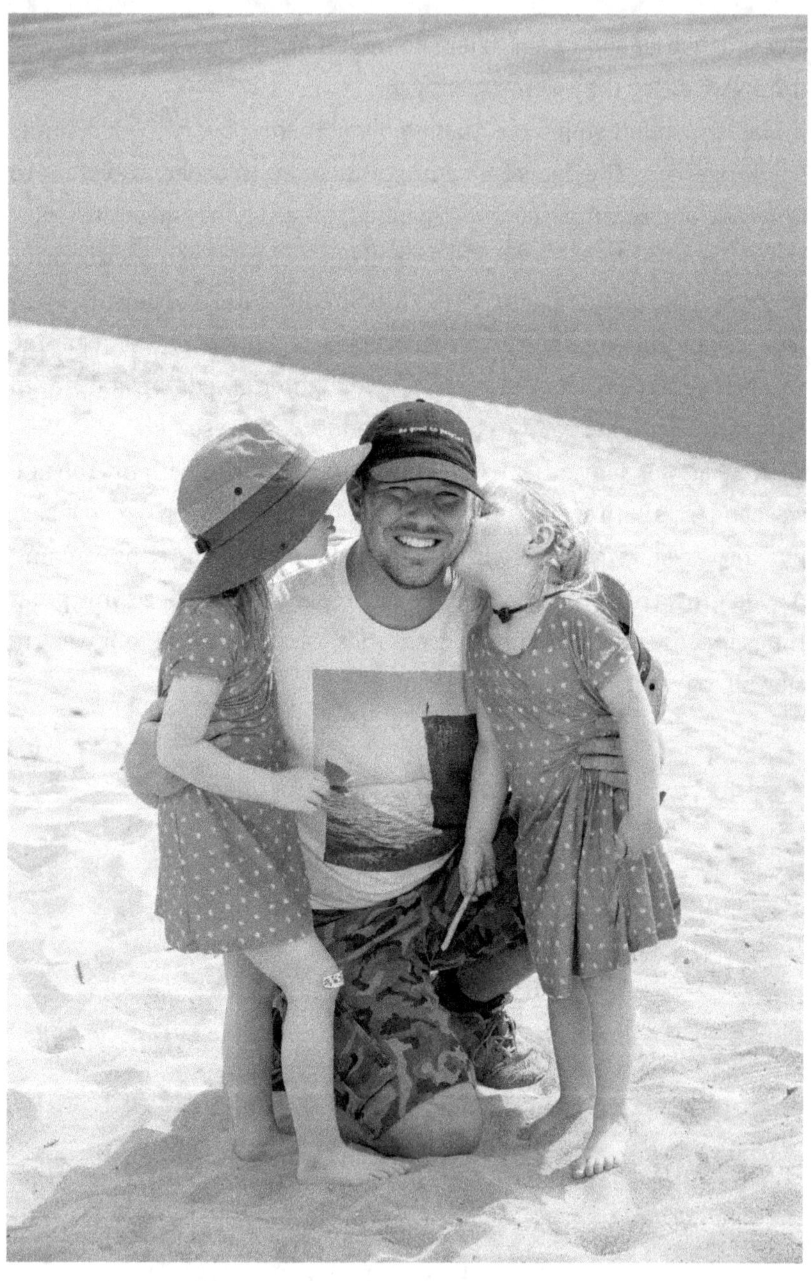

5

Chapter 5: Traditions

This is probably my favorite topic in this book. Since you now have become a single father household, create new family traditions at Dad's house. These are special things you do with your children at your home. These traditions can be simple or extravagant. What they can do is provide wonderful memories for your children that can last a lifetime. They may even hand some of these traditions down to their families. Family traditions bring your family members together emotionally and create a sense of belonging.

Traditions can provide stability. The kids know they're coming and look forward to them. Some traditions can involve cultural heritage or religion, but we're talking about traditions outside of those realms. Most family traditions involve activities that are fun. Your traditions can evolve over time. They can be as simple as movie night or game night. They can be weekend getaways, maybe camping and fishing. They could involve a sport. Superbowl family parties are great. My son and I try to do an annual golf competition with my brother and his son. You can create your own family traditions, but they should be fun, unique to your household, and memorable.

Of course, my favorite traditions are holiday celebrations. That is why this book is titled "Christmas at Dad's." These traditions often involve cultural, national, or religious rituals. They usually involve decorations, food, and other props. It could be a birthday tradition that you do every year on your child's birthday.

Going to a fireworks show every Fourth of July is one we try to do. I think everyone enjoys putting together costumes with their kids every Halloween. Carving the pumpkin together or having a pumpkin-carving competition between everyone. Thanksgiving is a big one. Every year, all over the country, families get together to enjoy a Thanksgiving feast. When you're divorced you usually have one at your house and the children have another one at their mother's house. If you're single, it's all yours. At my house, we would either go to Grandma or Grandpa's house, or one of my other siblings' houses. As we got older and people passed away, we started doing Thanksgiving at my house. Either I would cook a turkey or order everything made from a grocery store or specialty store. We always sit down at the big dining room table and gorge ourselves with delicious food. Always have to have black olives and claussen pickles though, tradition. Then we would have some dessert. We always had pumpkin pie and pecan pie. But another tradition is we always have a chocolate pie with whipped cream as well. No matter what though, everything is scheduled around the Cowboys game on Thanksgiving.

Now my favorite holiday is Christmas. I really go all out at Christmas. I want it to be memorable, fun, and exciting. When the kids were younger, their mother would also come over for Christmas. I think those were good memories for them. As the kids got older, and their mother and my life separated more, it would just be me and the kids. My daughter orders us all matching pajamas, including the kids' spouses. I spent all night wrapping gifts. Each kid would have twenty to thirty gifts. We would always go together to pick out the best tree, within budget, of course.

We would have a tree-decorating party. We would go shopping together and eat out together. This is such a bonding time of the year. You can really build some

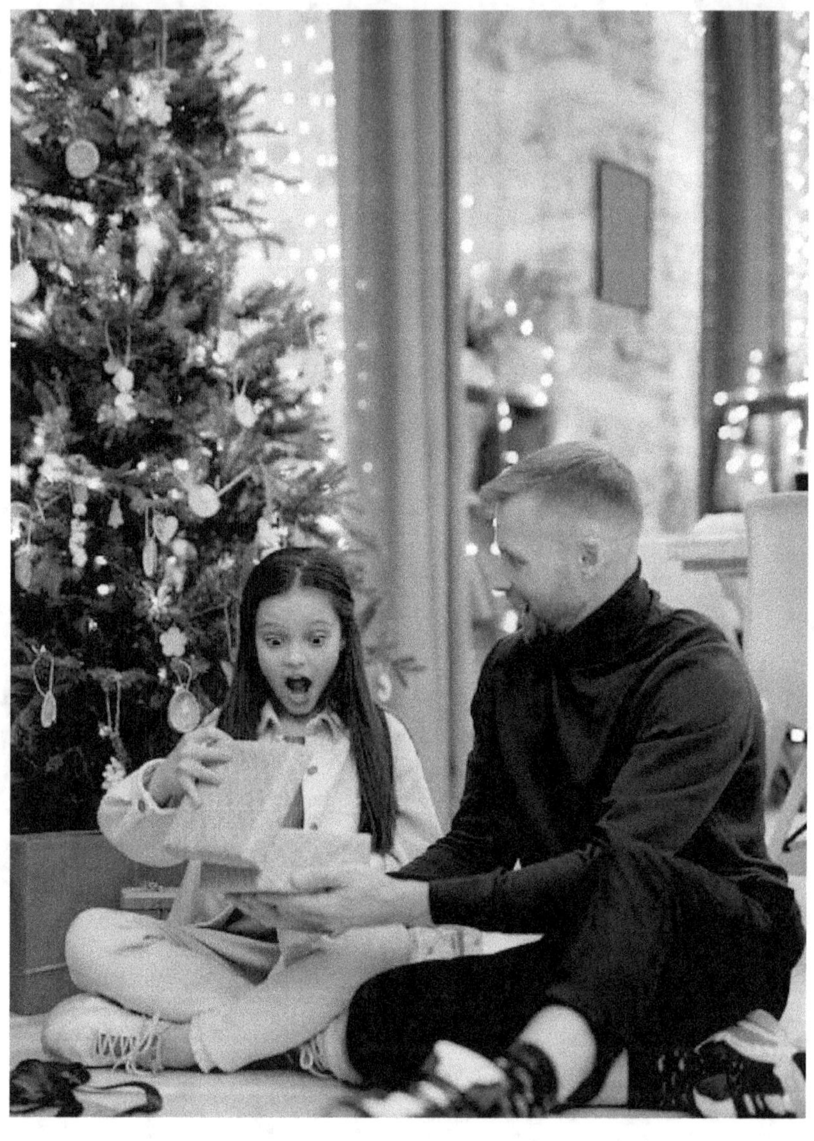

great memories together. When they were young, the kids and their mother and I would go to Christmas Eve service and then eat out at Benihana's. Now they do the Benihana's thing with their mother. I miss that but it's still a fond memory I have.

Then every Christmas morning, we would gather around the tree, pass out presents, and then take turns opening them. Now, I always had my kids write a Christmas wish list and things they needed, like clothes, shoes, whatever. I would budget out the same amount to spend on each child, and then I get as many things as I can on their list. However, I always try to get one surprise gift to each one every year that's really cool. One year was a drone, only $99 each. I would always find cool things at Sharper Image.

There were so many, I can't remember them all. The ideal though was to get them something that would wow them besides everything on their list. Make it more memorable. That's the whole idea of traditions. Things they will remember the rest of their lives that gave them joy.

I'm a sucker for Christmas. We still try to get together every Christmas at my house, but now there are a lot of other family factors involved. Again, the purpose of this book is to give you some suggestions that your children will really enjoy and not the same old crap you read in books.

One thing that has changed as a tradition over time with Christmas is we don't spend all our time out shopping anymore. Now it's Amazon, baby. These are the activities I remember with joy and I hope my children do as well. Build your own awesome, memorable traditions as a family. It will make a huge difference in raising your children.

6

Chapter 6: Going above and beyond

As a single father, one of the biggest challenges is taking care of your children while having to work and support the family financially. Start with arranging childcare. Whether you use a daycare, family members, or both. That's usually the case. You just want to make sure the kids are supervised and cared for while you're at work. You definitely don't want them to run wild. Coordinating with your ex can be very helpful here if you are divorced. If single, family members are the way to go, unless you can afford a nanny. I couldn't. You can divide childcare responsibilities like child drop-off and pickups with your ex. Watching the children if one of you has something important to do and it's your time with the kids is very helpful.

Identifying support systems is very important. We've already discussed family, but you can extend to friends or community organizations as well. Whatever is required to make sure your children are cared for. Absolutely, when you're home, spend as much time with them as possible. I think that goes without saying. Speak with your employer to let them know what's going on with your situation. This is very important. If you're a good employee and are valued, you would be amazed at how much your employer will understand. Being able to make my children's games and to go to other functions described earlier was a huge help from my employer. Sometimes having to take off because your child is sick or something happened to them was crucial and I was able to work that out with my employer as well. I believe you could do the same.

Remember to take some time for your self-care to manage the stress of holding down two jobs. Being a single father is also a job, but one I found very enjoyable. You can use exercise, yoga, stress release techniques, and counseling. All are good avenues. I myself exercised when I could. That helped me tremendously with stress. I also enjoyed playing golf when I had a chance to. Nothing like being out in nature, cursing your golf ball for not going straight.

Make sure you are taking care of your children's needs, even if it is going above and beyond. Try to listen to what they say, really listen to determine how they are feeling and what they need. Make sure your responses answer or help their needs. Talking with and listening to your children is probably the best thing you can do for their mental health. Compliment them often, especially if they are behaving correctly. Remember to be positive in raising your children. Do not criticize the child. Focus more on the behavior or mistakes. Provide structure to their lives, but always remember to hug and kiss them, show them how much you love them, and how much they mean to you.

If you help them build their self-esteem throughout their life, they will be better ready to cope with challenges throughout the rest of their lives.

Going above and beyond means you will do just about anything for your child and their needs. Responsive parenting is important. I experienced things like their mother sometimes could not get them what they needed. It might be something for school, a calculator, computer, instrument, clothes, or something they need for life. I was always willing to help out in those circumstances and it wasn't always easy. It may be something your ex needs to take care of the children, like having their car fixed so they could get around. Whatever I had to do, within reason, I was willing to do to raise my children. After all, their well being was and still is the most important thing to me.

As a parent later in life, you don't want to have any regrets about the experience of growing with your kids. Unfortunately, you probably will have some. Nobody's perfect, or at least I'm not. Every parent will make some mistakes throughout their life. No matter how much we love our children, we can sometimes unintentionally make wrong decisions in their upbringing. Just try to recognize their needs and set boundaries and consequences so they learn right from wrong.

Most of what I have experienced from talking to other parents, there are several regrets they have. Not spending enough quality time with their kids growing up, and then it's too late. Being too hard on them. I believe I was guilty of that at times. Some parents regret not providing enough financial support for their children. Don't let that bother you. Do what you can and what you can afford. Remember, there are a lot of things to do that don't cost money or cost very little money. Just provide what you can and be there for them.

I hear adults talk about not being present at some of their children's activities. Again, like games, recitals, father-daughter dances, and a plethora of other activities. Do your best to be there for your child. They know when you attend and when you're not there. It does make a big difference to them. They want you to share the joy and pride they are feeling. Definitely be there for important milestones or events. Things like kindergarten, middle school, and high school graduations. If your child goes to college, be there for them.

Parents many times regret not having boundaries for their kids as they grow up. This often leads to behavioral issues and other problems later in life. Make sure that is a part of their upbringing: rules and boundaries. That will make your child a well-balanced adult. This is one of my regrets. I too often was a big child with my kids and wanted to be their best friend as well. It's important that parents lead by example. It's not "do as I say, not as I do." This is an old adage I often hear parents say. Terrible example for your children. Just make sure you listen to them and communicate with them respectfully.

Did you know that according to the US Census Bureau from 2022, 18.3 million children across America live without a father in their home. That is one in four children. That's ridiculous. Don't abandon your children and start over someplace else. You can still start over, just do it with your children. They need you. Don't have regrets later in life that not only affect your kids, but you as well. Being a parent is challenging and comes with a wide range of emotions. It's important to recognize your mistakes and learn from them when you are prioritizing your children's needs. Communicate with them, you can create a healthy environment for them to grow up in. They will be happy, optimistic, and well-adjusted adults.

7

Conclusion

Conclusion:

This is hopefully a good resource single and divorced fathers can use to navigate their children's upbringing. Just do the absolute best you can to raise your children and be there for them. Hopefully they will grow up to be happy and well-adjusted adults, and have families of their own. You will be giving them a better chance to do so.They can pass down some of the traditions you and them created growing together.

All three of my children are now married and are starting their own families. I just had my first grand-daughter, little Momo. Can't love her enough. Now I have to learn how to be a grandfather. That should be exciting. Unfortunately, this story has somewhat of an imperfect ending. I spend wonderful times with my son and his wife, my youngest daughter, her husband, and little Momo, but I no longer have communications with my eldest daughter. She lives far away and doesn't want to be part of my life anymore. I tried for a couple of years to regain a relationship, but it just hasn't worked out. I still love her and her husband and maybe one day, that will have a happy ending as well.

As I have said before, nobody's perfect. Most people in the world today would say there's something they would like to change about their lives and I fall into that category. I did try my best to bring my children up properly with love and I will continue to keep channels open for my daughter. Hopefully my relationship with my daughter will change for the better in the future. The rest of us are very happy together and spend as much time as we can together.

Fathers, enjoy life with your children and good luck!

If you found this book helpful or enjoyed it, I would be very appreciative if you would leave a favorable review for the book on Amazon! Thank you!

Resources:

Shipe, S. L., Ayer, L., & Guastaferro, K. (2021). American Single father homes: a growing public health priority. *American Journal of Public Health*, 112(1), 21–23. https://doi.org/10.2105/ajph.2021.306591

The Annie E. Casey Foundation. (2024, April 6). *Child Well-Being in*

Single-Parent families. Retrieved October 26, 2024, from https://www.a ecf.org/blog/child-well-being-in-single-parent-families?gad_source =1&gclid=CjoKCQjwpvK4BhDUARIsADHt9sTJTGotJj5M7oVGqXtMWa-C _2yBvV6N6S0Z38gg1UKluHq7ki8pb6UaAo_DEALw_wcB

Buckley, C. K. (2013). Co-Parenting after Divorce: Opportunities and challenges. In *Clinical Science Insights*. The Family Institute at Northwestern University. Retrieved October 26, 2024, from https://ww w.family-institute.org/sites/default/files/pdfs/csi_buckley_co-parenti ng_after_divorce.pdf

Family means. (2024). *What are the effects of divorce on children? | FamilyMeans*. Family Means. Retrieved October 26, 2024, from https://w ww.familymeans.org/effects-of-divorce-on-children.html

Lomantini, A., & Lomantini, A. (2023, July 31). Navigating Divorce with Kids: Words & Actions to Avoid. *Kids in the Middle – Counseling for Children, Parents & Families*. Retrieved October 26, 2024, from https://ki dsinthemiddle.org/navigating-divorce-with-kids-words-actions-to-a void/

Eritchie. (2022, January 20). *8 Ways to Strengthen a Parent-Child Relationship | Family Services*. Family Services. Retrieved October 26, 2024, from https://www.familyservicesnew.org/news/8-ways-to-stre ngthen-a-parent-child-relationship/

Nielsen, V. a. P. B. A. (2023, March 31). *Creating your child's childhood*. Big Abilities. Retrieved October 26, 2024, from https://bigabilities.com/ 2018/10/09/creating-your-childs-childhood/

Holmes, M. (2022, August 9). You're trying to give your kids an amazing childhood. How much will they remember? *HuffPost*. https://w ww.huffpost.com/entry/how-much-do-kids-remember_l_62e949bce 4b006483aa1bc3d

Thatcher, T. & Highland Springs Specialty Clinic. (2024). *Highland*

Springs Specialty Clinic – The top ten benefits of spending time with family. Highland Springs Specialty Clinic. Retrieved October 26, 2024, from https://highlandspringsclinic.org/the-top-ten-benefits-of-spending-time-with-family

Russell, A. (2024, July). *28 Fun and meaningful family traditions to treasure forever.* Remento. Retrieved October 26, 2024, from https://www.remento.co/journal/fun-and-meaningful-family-traditions-to-treasure-forever

Sanford Health News & Parenting Services. (2022, December 6). *Responsive parenting: 3 steps to meet your child's needs.* Sanford Health News. Retrieved October 26, 2024, from https://news.sanfordhealth.org/parenting/responsive-parenting-3-steps-to-meet-your-childs-needs/

Bokhari, S. (2023, February 13). *Top 7 Parental Regrets & Guilts and their Solutions.* Linkedin. Retrieved October 26, 2024, from https://www.linkedin.com/pulse/top-7-parental-regrets-guilts-solutions-saleem-bokhari**Conclusion:**